# FLEXIBILTY REDUCE PAIN

*"Flexibility Revolution: Transforming Pain into Comfort"*

**By**
**Ellie Grace**

# TABLE OF CONTENT

# 4

## Introduction:

Adaptability assumes a vital part in the mind boggling dance of human development. Past its tasteful allure in smooth stretches and distortions, adaptability fills in as a foundation in the domain of torment decrease and the executives. This powerful transaction among adaptability and agony isn't only hypothetical however established profoundly in the physiological components of the human body.

In this investigation, we set out on an excursion diving into the cooperative connection among adaptability and torment decrease. Torment, whether intense or ongoing, appears as a sign of trouble inside the body, frequently coming from solid strain, joint firmness, or primary irregular characteristics. On the other hand, adaptability goes about as a strong counteract ant, offering freedom from the shackles of torment by reestablishing portability, improving flow, and cultivating strength inside the outer muscle framework.

As we cross through the complexities of adaptability and its significant effect on torment decrease, we unwind the logical underpinnings, dig into commonsense procedures, and uncover the extraordinary power that exists in the domain of psyche body association. Through this excursion, we expect to furnish you with the information, devices, and bits of knowledge important to embrace adaptability as a foundation of your aggravation the executive's routine, engaging you to open an existence of more prominent solace, essentialness, and opportunity.

# Chapter 1
## Understanding Pain

Torment is a widespread encounter, an inborn part of human life that rises above social, social, and geological limits. A complex peculiarity appears in horde structures, from the intense sting of a paper slice to the relentless hurt of an ongoing condition. Regardless of its pervasiveness, torment stays a complex and frequently misconstrued idea, enveloping both physiological and mental aspects. In this exhaustive investigation, we attempt to disentangle the complex woven artwork of agony, digging into its systems, characterizations, discernments, and suggestions for human wellbeing and prosperity.

At its center, torment fills in as a crucial caution framework, making the body aware of expected dangers and provoking defensive reactions. This nociceptive flagging, started by particular nerve receptors known as nociceptors, communicates data about tissue harm or injury to the focal sensory system (CNS), where it is handled and deciphered. The view of torment not entirely set in stone by the seriousness of tissue harm but at the same time is impacted by a variety of variables, including close to home state, previous encounters, social foundation, and mental examination.

One of the key qualifications in understanding torment lies in its arrangement into intense and persistent classifications. Intense torment commonly emerges out of nowhere because of tissue injury or injury and is portrayed by a sharp, limited vibe that fills in as an advance notice signal. Conversely, persistent torment endures past the normal recuperating time and is in many cases joined by a large number of physical, profound, and social outcomes. Persistent agony can come from different sources, including hidden ailments like joint inflammation, fibromyalgia, or neuropathy, as well as psychosocial factors like pressure, nervousness, and despondency.

The instruments basic agony insight are mind boggling and complex, including multifaceted collaborations between the sensory system, insusceptible framework, endocrine framework, and mental variables. Key to this cycle is the idea of nociception, the brain encoding and handling of poisonous improvements inside the CNS. Nociceptive torment, which emerges from enactment of nociceptors in light of tissue harm or injury, addresses an essential part of the body's safeguard systems. This kind of aggravation is regularly intense in nature and fills in as an advance notice sign to make the individual aware of expected hurt.

Be that as it may, torment insight still up in the air by nociceptive info but at the same time is significantly impacted by a heap of variables, including mental, profound, and social elements. The bio psychosocial model of torment stresses the exchange between natural, mental, and social variables in forming the singular experience of agony. As indicated by this model, torment isn't simply a tactile peculiarity yet a perplexing, multi-layered experience that is impacted by a huge number of variables, including previous encounters, convictions assumptions, and social standards.

Mental elements, like consideration, assumption, and discernment, assume a critical part in molding the emotional experience of torment. For instance, people who catastrophism or amplify the seriousness of their aggravation might encounter uplifted degrees of misery and inability, while the individuals who utilize versatile survival methods, like care or mental rebuilding, may encounter more noteworthy torment resistance and flexibility. Likewise, close to home variables, including tension, sadness, and stress, can adjust torment insight through their consequences for synapse frameworks, neuroendocrine capability, and safe capability.

Social elements, like social help, financial status, and social convictions, additionally apply a huge impact on torment insight and the board. Social help has been displayed to cushion against the adverse consequence of agony on physical and mental prosperity, while social seclusion or saw shame can compound agony and add to handicap. Social convictions and standards encompassing agony can shape people's mentalities toward torment articulation, help-chasing conduct, and treatment inclinations.

Notwithstanding nociceptive agony, which emerges from actuation of nociceptors because of tissue harm or injury there are other unmistakable sorts of agony that emerge from brokenness or harm to the sensory system itself. Neuropathic torment, for instance, results from injury or brokenness of the fringe or focal sensory system and is portrayed by strange sensations like copying, shivering, or shooting torment. Instances of conditions related with neuropathic torment incorporate diabetic neuropathy, post herpetic neuralgia, and spinal string injury.

One more classification of agony, known as fiery agony, emerges from actuation of the safe framework because of tissue injury or contamination. Incendiary agony is portrayed by redness, enlarging, intensity, and delicacy at the site of injury and is intervened by fiery go between like prostaglandins, cytokines, and bradykinin. Instances of conditions related with provocative torment incorporate rheumatoid joint pain, incendiary inside infection, and intense injury or injury.

Psychogenic agony, additionally alluded to as psychosomatic agony or somatoform torment jumble, is torment that isn't owing to any recognizable actual reason however is accepted to be impacted by mental factors like pressure, uneasiness, or misery. Psychogenic agony is many times depicted as diffuse, ambiguous, and inadequately limited and might be related with other substantial side effects like weakness, sleep deprivation, or gastrointestinal pain. Instances of conditions related with psychogenic torment incorporate fibromyalgia, peevish gut disorder, and strain cerebral pains.

The impression of torment is intrinsically emotional differing generally from one individual to another and impacted by a large number of variables, including organic, mental, and social elements. Torment power, term, and quality can change extraordinarily contingent upon individual contrasts in torment edges, torment resilience, and agony survival techniques. Besides, social convictions, accepted practices, and previous encounters can shape how agony is deciphered, communicated, and answered.

In spite of its emotional nature, torment is a substantial reality for a large number of people around the world addressing a critical weight on physical, profound, and social prosperity. Constant torment, specifically, represents a significant test for medical care frameworks, influencing roughly one-fifth of the worldwide populace and representing a significant piece of medical services uses. The financial expenses of constant agony are faltering, incorporating direct clinical expenses, roundabout costs like lost efficiency and handicap, and immaterial costs like lessened personal satisfaction and mental pain.

Considering the gigantic weight of agony on people, networks, and social orders, there is a squeezing need for exhaustive ways to deal with torment the board that address the complex idea of torment and its fundamental systems. This requires a shift away from the conventional biomedical model of torment, which centers exclusively on the physiological parts of agony and underscores pharmacological mediations, toward a more
All encompassing, bio psychosocial model that perceives the interconnectedness of natural, mental, and social elements in molding the aggravation experience.

Such a methodology requires a multidisciplinary way to deal with torment the board that coordinates pharmacological intercessions with reciprocal and elective treatments, for example, non-intrusive treatment, mental social treatment, care based pressure decrease, needle therapy, and back rub treatment. Besides, endeavors to address the social determinants of wellbeing, like neediness, imbalance, and social rejection, are fundamental for lessening aberrations in torment care and further developing results for weak populaces.

All in all, torment is a mind boggling, diverse peculiarity that envelops both physiological and mental aspects. Grasping the systems, arrangements, insights, and ramifications of torment is fundamental for creating successful techniques for torment the executives and working on the personal satisfaction for people living with torment. By taking on a comprehensive, bio psychosocial way to deal with torment the executives that tends to the interconnectedness of natural, mental, and social elements, we can make ready toward a future where torment isn't just persevered however eased, moderated, and eventually rose above.

# Chapter 2
# The Science of Flexibility

Adaptability is a basic part of actual wellness, including the capacity of muscles and joints to travel through a full scope of movement without limitation or uneasiness. It assumes a critical part in different exercises of day to day living, sports execution, and injury counteraction. While many individuals partner adaptability with exercises, for example, yoga or vaulting, a quality is pertinent to people of any age and wellness levels. In this complete investigation, we dig into the science behind adaptability, looking at its physiological systems, benefits, and reasonable ramifications for wellbeing and execution.

## Physiology of Adaptability

Still up in the air by a few variables, including muscle length, joint construction, connective tissue versatility, and neuromuscular coordination. At the phone level, adaptability is affected by the properties of muscle tissue, explicitly the game plan of contractile proteins inside muscle strands. The essential protein engaged with muscle constriction is actin, which structures slight fibers, and myosin, which frames thick fibers. These fibers slide past one another during muscle compression, considering development to happen.

Muscle adaptability is likewise impacted by the versatility of connective tissues like ligaments, tendons, and belt. Ligaments append muscles to bones, while tendons associate unresolved issues bones, giving steadiness and backing to joints. Sash is a thick, sinewy connective tissue that encompasses muscles, bones, and organs, giving primary uprightness and working with development. The versatility of these tissues permits them to stretch and backlash in light of pressure, subsequently adding to generally speaking adaptability.

Neuromuscular coordination assumes a significant part in deciding adaptability by directing the enactment and unwinding of muscles during development. The sensory system conveys messages to muscle filaments by means of engine neurons, setting off muscle withdrawals and controlling development designs. Adaptability preparing can work on neuromuscular coordination by upgrading the correspondence between the sensory system and muscles, bringing about smoother, more productive development designs.

## Advantages of Adaptability

Adaptability preparing offers a great many advantages for both physical and mental prosperity. A portion of the key advantages include:

## *Expanded Scope of Movement:*

Adaptability preparing can work on joint versatility and scope of movement, considering more prominent opportunity of development in exercises of everyday living and sports execution.

## Injury Avoidance:

Keeping up with ideal adaptability can assist with forestalling wounds by diminishing the gamble of muscle strains, tendon injuries, and joint disengagements. Further developed adaptability permits tissues to ingest and disperse powers all the more actually, decreasing the probability of abuse wounds.

## Upgraded Execution:

Adaptability preparing can work on athletic execution by empowering competitors to move all the more proficiently and successfully. Expanded scope of movement considers more prominent power age, deftness, and coordination, prompting further developed sports execution.

## Relief from discomfort:

Adaptability activities can assist with easing muscle strain and firmness, decreasing uneasiness and advancing unwinding. Extending can likewise animate the arrival of endorphins, regular agony alleviating synthetic compounds created by the body.

## Further developed Stance:

Adaptability preparing can further develop pose by extending tight muscles and diminishing awkward nature between contradicting muscle gatherings. Better stance can lighten stress on the spine and joints, decreasing the gamble of outer muscle torment and injury.

## *Stress Decrease:*

Adaptability practices advance unwinding and stress help by empowering profound breathing, care, and body mindfulness. Extending can assist with quieting the sensory system, diminish muscle strain, and advance a feeling of prosperity.

# Standards of Adaptability Preparing

Powerful adaptability preparing includes sticking to specific standards to augment the advantages while limiting the gamble of injury. A few key standards include:

## *Warm-up:*

Continuously start adaptability preparing with a careful get ready to increment blood stream to muscles, raise center internal heat level, and set up the body for extending. Dynamic developments, for example, arm circles, leg swings, and middle turns are phenomenal warm-up works out.

## Steady Movement:

Continuously increment the power and term of extending practices after some time to try not to overextend or stressing muscles. Begin with delicate stretches and step by step increment the force as adaptability moves along.

## Hold and Relax:

Hold each stretch for 15-30 seconds and spotlight on profound, cadenced breathing to work with unwinding and discharge strain. Try not to bob or snapping developments, which can expand the gamble of injury.

## Equilibrium and Evenness:

Keep up with equilibrium and balance between restricting muscle bunches by extending the two sides of the body similarly. Center around extending tight muscles while keeping up  with adaptability in restricting muscles to forestall irregular characteristics and lessen the gamble of injury.

## Consistency:

Integrate adaptability preparing into your standard
 Work-out daily schedule and perform extending practices somewhere around 2-3 times each week to keep up with adaptability and forestall loss of scope of movement.

## *Variety:*

Remember an assortment of extending methods for your adaptability normal, like static extending, dynamic extending, and proprioceptive neuromuscular help (PNF) extending, to target different muscle gatherings and work on generally adaptability.

# Down to earth Uses of Adaptability Preparing

Adaptability preparing can be integrated into various exercises and settings, making it open to people of any age and wellness levels. A few pragmatic uses of adaptability preparing include:

## *Work out schedules:*

Incorporate adaptability practices as a feature of a balanced work out regime to work on generally versatility, decrease the gamble of injury, and upgrade practice execution. Integrate extending practices into your warm-up and chill off schedules to set up the body for action and advance recuperation.

## *Sports Molding:*

Integrate sport-explicit adaptability practices into preparing projects to work on athletic execution and diminish the gamble of sports-related wounds. Center around extending tight muscles and joints that are inclined to injury in your picked sport,  like hamstrings in sprinters or shoulders in swimmers.

## Rehabilitation:

Use adaptability practices as a component of a restoration program to work on joint portability, decrease torment, and reestablish capability following injury or medical procedure. Progressively once again introduce extending practices as endured to forestall solidness and advance mending.

## Work environment Health:

Advance adaptability preparing as a component of a work environment health program to decrease the gamble of outer muscle wounds and further develop representative efficiency and spirit. Urge representatives to enjoy customary stretch reprieves over the course of the day to battle the adverse consequences of delayed sitting and dreary movement.

## Maturing Populace:

Offer adaptability preparing programs custom fitted to the requirements of more established grown-ups to further develop portability, diminish fall hazard, and upgrade personal satisfaction. Center around delicate extending practices that target tight muscles and joints ordinarily impacted by maturing, like hips, shoulders, and spine.

# End

All in all, adaptability preparing is a fundamental part of actual wellness that offers various advantages for wellbeing, execution, and by and large prosperity. By grasping the physiological systems basic adaptability, as well as its useful applications in different settings, people can enhance their adaptability preparing schedules to accomplish their wellness objectives and work on their personal satisfaction. Whether you're a competitor taking a stab at max operation, a stationary individual looking to further develop versatility, or a more established grown-up planning to keep up with freedom, adaptability preparing can assume a critical part in assisting you with arriving at your maximum capacity and partake in an existence of wellbeing and imperativeness.

# Chapter 3
# Benefits of Flexibility

Adaptability, frequently neglected for strength or cardiovascular wellness, is a foundation of generally actual wellbeing and prosperity. Characterized as the capacity of muscles and joints to travel through a full scope of movement without agony or uneasiness, adaptability assumes a pivotal part in different parts of day to day existence, sports execution, and injury counteraction. In this exhaustive investigation, we dig into the large number of advantages related with adaptability preparing, analyzing its effect on actual wellbeing, athletic execution, and mental prosperity.

## Actual Medical advantages

Further developed Scope of Movement: Adaptability preparing improves joint portability and scope of movement, taking into consideration smoother, more smooth motion designs. This expanded adaptability can further develop act, lessen firmness, and lighten uneasiness related with exercises of day to day living.

## *Injury Avoidance:*

Keeping up with ideal adaptability can assist with forestalling wounds by decreasing the gamble of muscle strains, tendon injuries, and joint separations. By permitting tissues to assimilate and scatter powers all the more successfully, adaptability preparing can moderate the effect of abrupt developments or outside influences.

## Upgraded Muscle Capability:

Adaptability preparing advances ideal muscle capability by guaranteeing that  muscles can protract and contract through their full scope of movement. This superior muscle capability can improve muscle strength, perseverance, and power, prompting better execution in sports and exercises.

## Joint Wellbeing and Life span:

Adaptability preparing upholds joint wellbeing and life span by advancing appropriate arrangement, diminishing mileage on joint surfaces, and forestalling the improvement of degenerative circumstances like osteoarthritis. By keeping up with ideal joint capability, adaptability preparing can assist with protecting versatility and freedom as we age.

## Help with discomfort:

Adaptability activities can assist with mitigating muscle pressure, solidness, and distress, diminishing the impression of torment and advancing unwinding. Extending can invigorate the arrival of endorphins, normal agony easing synthetics created by the body, giving alleviation from persistent torment conditions.

# Athletic Execution Advantages

## *Expanded Spryness and Coordination:*

Adaptability preparing further develops deftness and coordination by upgrading neuromuscular control and proprioception. Competitors with more noteworthy adaptability can move all the more proficiently and actually, taking a different path rapidly and responding to unusual developments effortlessly.

## *Upgraded Power and Strength:*

Adaptability preparing supplements strength preparing by permitting muscles to produce more noteworthy power through a full scope of movement. This expanded power and strength can convert into further developed execution in unstable developments like hopping, running, and lifting.

## *Diminished Hazard of Sports Wounds:*

Adaptability preparing diminishes the gamble of Sports-related wounds by working on joint versatility, muscle adaptability, and tissue flexibility. Competitors with more noteworthy adaptability are less inclined to encounter abuse wounds or strains because of unnecessary pressure or confined development.

## Further developed Recuperation and Recovery:

Adaptability practices advance quicker recuperation and recovery by expanding blood stream to muscles, lessening muscle irritation, and advancing unwinding. Extending can assist with flushing out metabolic byproducts like lactic corrosive and advance the conveyance of oxygen and supplements to muscle tissues.

## Upgraded Execution Potential:

Adaptability preparing improves execution potential by tending to irregular characteristics, deviations, and constraints that might upset athletic execution. By recognizing and tending to areas of snugness or shortcoming, competitors can open their full actual potential and accomplish maximized operation.

## Mental Prosperity Advantages

## Stress Decrease:

Adaptability preparing advances unwinding and stress help by empowering profound breathing, care, and body mindfulness. Extending activities can assist with quieting the sensory system, lessen muscle pressure, and advance a feeling of quiet and prosperity.

## Improved Psyche Body Association:

Adaptability preparing upgrades the brain body association by cultivating consciousness of actual sensations, developments, and arrangement. This uplifted mindfulness can advance care, fixation, and mindfulness, prompting worked on mental clearness and concentration.

## Further developed Mind-set and Energy Levels:

Adaptability practices animate the arrival of endorphins Synapses that advance sensations of joy and prosperity. Customary extending can help mind-set, mitigate side effects of misery and nervousness, and increment energy levels by decreasing sensations of exhaustion and torpidity.

## Improved Unwinding and Rest Quality:

Adaptability preparing advances unwinding and further developed rest quality by diminishing muscle strain advancing actual unwinding, and quieting the psyche. Extending before sleep time can assist with setting up the body and brain for relaxing rest, prompting a more helpful and reviving night's rest.

## *Expanded Fearlessness and Confidence:*

Adaptability preparing helps fearlessness and confidence by encouraging a feeling of achievement, dominance, and self-viability. As people progress in their adaptability practice and accomplish their objectives, they gain a more noteworthy identity certainty and confidence in their capacities.

## **Pragmatic Utilizations of Adaptability Preparing**

Adaptability preparing can be integrated into different settings and exercises to receive its heap rewards. A few down to earth utilizations of adaptability preparing include:

## *Work out schedules:*

Incorporate adaptability practices as a component of a balanced work out regime to work on generally versatility, diminish the gamble of injury, and upgrade practice execution. Integrate extending practices into warm-up and chill off schedules to set up the body for action and advance recuperation.

## *Sports Molding:*

 Integrate sport-explicit adaptability practices into preparing projects to work on athletic execution and decrease the gamble of sports-related wounds.
 Center around extending tight muscles and joints that are inclined to injury in your picked sport, like hamstrings in sprinters or shoulders in swimmers.

## *Rehabilitation:*

Use adaptability practices as a feature of a recovery program to work on joint versatility, diminish torment, and reestablish capability following injury or medical procedure. Steadily once again introduce extending practices as endured to forestall firmness and advance recuperating.

## *Work environment Health:*

 Advance adaptability preparing as a feature of a working environment health program to diminish the gamble of outer muscle wounds and further develop worker efficiency and spirit. Urge workers to enjoy ordinary stretch reprieves over the course of the day to battle the adverse consequences of drawn out sitting and dull movement.

## *Maturing Populace:*

Offer adaptability preparing programs custom-made to the necessities of more seasoned grown-ups to further develop portability, lessen fall chance, and improve personal satisfaction. Center around delicate extending practices that target tight muscles and joints normally impacted by maturing, like hips, shoulders, and spine.

# End

All in all, adaptability preparing offers many advantages for actual wellbeing, athletic execution, and mental prosperity. By integrating adaptability practices into your normal daily schedule and taking on an all-encompassing way to deal with wellness and wellbeing, you can upgrade your adaptability, work on your general wellbeing and execution, and improve your personal satisfaction. Whether you're a competitor taking a stab at maximized execution, a wellness fan trying to further develop versatility, or a singular hoping to diminish pressure and improve prosperity, adaptability preparing can assume a urgent part in assisting you with accomplishing your objectives and carry on with a better, more dynamic way of life.

# Chapter 4
# Flexibility Techniques

Adaptability is a vital part of by and large wellness and wellbeing, adding to further developed execution in proactive tasks, diminished chance of injury, and upgraded personal satisfaction. Adaptability strategies include a large number of activities and techniques intended to work on joint portability, muscle versatility, and scope of movement. In this extensive aide, we investigate different adaptability procedures, including static extending, dynamic extending, proprioceptive neuromuscular assistance (PNF), froth rolling, yoga, and Pilates, looking at their advantages, applications, and commonsense contemplations for integrating them into your wellness schedule.

## Static Extending

Static extending is maybe the most notable and broadly rehearsed type of adaptability work out. It includes standing firm on a stretch in a fixed foothold for a set term, ordinarily going from 15 to 60 seconds. Static extending targets explicit muscle gatherings and means to step by step stretch tight muscles, work on joint versatility, and increment scope of movement. A few vital contemplations for static extending include:

## *Technique:*

Perform static stretches gradually and delicately, trying not to skip or yanking developments that can cause muscle strain or injury. Center around keeping up with great stance and arrangement all through the stretch, and inhale profoundly and equally to work with unwinding.

## *Duration:*

Hold every static stretch for 15 to 60 seconds, intending to arrive at a mark of gentle inconvenience or pressure, however not torment. Try not to drive into a stretch too forcefully, as this can set off the stretch reflex and prompt muscles to fix as opposed to unwind.

## *Frequency:*

Integrate static extending into your wellness routine something like 2 to 3 times each week, in a perfect world after an exhaustive warm-up or toward the finish of an exercise when muscles are warm and flexible. Intend to extend all significant muscle gatherings, zeroing in on areas of snugness or limitation.

## Dynamic Extending

Dynamic extending includes moving the body through a full scope of movement in a controlled way, utilizing force and energy to build adaptability and portability progressively. Dissimilar to static extending, which centers on standing firm on a stretch in a fixed situation, dynamic extending stresses liquid, nonstop developments that imitate the activities of sports or exercises. A few vital contemplations for dynamic extending include:

## *Technique:*

Perform dynamic stretches in a sluggish, controlled way zeroing in on smooth, musical developments that continuously expansion in power and scope of movement. Focus on legitimate structure and arrangement, and keep away from jerky or ballistic developments that can strain muscles or joints.

## *Variety:*

Integrate an assortment of dynamic stretches into your warm-up everyday practice, focusing on various muscle gatherings and development designs. Incorporate developments, for example, leg swings, arm circles, middle winds, and rush varieties to set up the body for the particular requests of your exercise or movement.

## *Specificity:*

Pick dynamic stretches that are pertinent to your game or action, zeroing in on developments that copy the activities and biomechanics of your picked action. For instance, assuming you're a sprinter, incorporate dynamic stretches that stress hip flexion, expansion, and pivot to set up the muscles and joints for running.

# Proprioceptive Neuromuscular Assistance (PNF)

Proprioceptive neuromuscular help (PNF) is an extending procedure that consolidates detached extending with isometric constrictions to build adaptability and scope of movement. PNF extending normally includes an accomplice or a prop, for example, an opposition band or dependability ball, to work with more profound extending and more noteworthy increases in adaptability. A few vital contemplations for PNF extending include:

## Technique:

PNF extending commonly includes three stages: uninvolved extending, isometric constriction, and inactive extending. Begin by inactively extending the objective muscle to its end scope of movement, then, at that point, play out an isometric compression by pushing against an accomplice or opposition band for 5 to 10 seconds. At last, loosen up the muscle and latently stretch it once more, planning to accomplish a more noteworthy scope of movement.

## Accomplice or Prop:

PNF extending frequently requires an accomplice to help with the extending or a prop, for example, an obstruction band or solidness ball to give opposition and backing. Discuss obviously with your accomplice and guarantee that they grasp the appropriate procedure and force of the stretch.

## *Safety:*

Practice alert while performing PNF extending, particularly on the off chance that you're new to the procedure or working with an accomplice. Begin with delicate stretches and step by step increment the force and length as endured. Try not to drive into agony or inconvenience, and pay attention to your body's signs to abstain from overextending or injury.

# Froth Rolling

Froth rolling, otherwise called self-Myofascial discharge, is a self-rub procedure that utilizes a barrel shaped froth roller to apply strain to tight or limited areas of muscle and connective tissue. Froth moving aides discharge attachments, bunches, and trigger focuses in the muscles, further developing blood stream, diminishing muscle strain, and improving adaptability. A few critical contemplations for froth rolling include:

## *Technique:*

Utilize slow, controlled developments to move the froth roller along the length of the muscle, stopping on areas of snugness or inconvenience. Apply delicate to direct strain to the muscle, keeping away from unnecessary power or moving straight over hard prominences or joints.

## *Frequency:*

Integrate froth moving into your warm-up or chill off daily schedule or as a feature of a recuperation meeting after extraordinary activity or movement. Intend to move each significant muscle bunch for 1 to 2 minutes, zeroing in on areas of snugness or limitation.

## *Variety:*

Try different things with various froth moving methods and procedures, like moving in numerous headings, utilizing various sizes and densities of froth rollers, or consolidating dynamic developments, for example, shaking or bending while at the same time rolling. Find what turns out best for your body and explicit areas of snugness or limitation.

## Yoga

Yoga is a centuries-old practice that consolidates actual stances, breath control, and care contemplation to advance physical, mental, and profound prosperity. Yoga underlines adaptability, strength, equilibrium, and unwinding, making it an optimal practice for working on generally versatility and scope of movement. A few vital contemplations for yoga practice include:

## Postures:

Yoga stances, or asana, are intended to extend and reinforce the muscles, joints, and connective tissues of the body. Rehearsing an assortment of yoga stances can further develop adaptability, portability, and soundness all through the body, advancing better stance, arrangement, and development designs.

## Breathe Mindfulness:

Breath mindfulness, or pranayama, is a fundamental part of yoga practice that helps quiet the psyche, decrease pressure, and upgrade focus. Coordinate your breath with development during yoga work on, breathing in profoundly as you venture into a stretch and breathing out completely as you discharge strain and unwind.

## Care Contemplation:

Yoga consolidates care contemplation procedures, for example, zeroed in consideration on the breath, body check, and directed symbolism to advance unwinding, stress decrease, and mental lucidity. Develop a feeling of present-second mindfulness during yoga work on, permitting contemplations and interruptions to condemn or connection.

# Pilates

Pilates is a brain body practice framework created by Joseph Pilates in the mid twentieth century that spotlights on fortifying the center muscles, further developing stance, and upgrading in general body mindfulness and control. Pilate's practices accentuate accuracy, arrangement, and breathe control, making them ideal for further developing adaptability and versatility. A few critical contemplations for Pilates practice include:

## *Center Dependability:*

Pilate's practices underscore center soundness and control, focusing on the profound muscles of the mid-region, back, and pelvis. By fortifying the center muscles and further developing arrangement, Pilates can improve generally body mindfulness, stance, and development effectiveness.

## *Practical Development Examples:*

Pilate's practices center on useful development designs that impersonate exercises of everyday living, like bowing, contorting, coming to, and lifting. By rehearsing these development designs in a controlled and careful way, Pilates can further develop adaptability, portability, and strength all through the body.

## *Breathe Combination:*

Pilates accentuates breath mix with development empowering profound, diaphragmatic breathing to help and improve the viability of each activity. Coordinate your breath with development during Pilates work on, breathing in to get ready for a development and breathing out to start and finish the development.

# End

All in all, adaptability procedures offer a different exhibit of activities and techniques for working on joint versatility, muscle flexibility, and scope of movement. By integrating static extending, dynamic extending, PNF extending, froth rolling, yoga, or Pilates into your wellness schedule, you can upgrade adaptability, diminish the gamble of injury, and work on generally speaking actual wellbeing and prosperity. Try different things with various procedures, find what turns out best for your body and explicit requirements, and partake in the advantages of expanded adaptability, versatility, and imperativeness in your day to day existence.

# Chapter 5
# Mind-Body Connection

The psyche and body have for quite some time been seen as unmistakable substances, with independent areas of impact and control.  Notwithstanding, arising research in fields like brain science, neuroscience, and integrative medication has uncovered the significant interconnectedness of these apparently discrete parts of human experience. The brain body association alludes to the mind boggling transaction among mental and actual wellbeing, wherein contemplations, feelings, convictions, and perspectives can significantly impact physiological cycles as well as the other way around. In this extensive investigation, we dive into the complex idea of the psyche body association, analyzing its suggestions for wellbeing, health, and comprehensive recuperating.

## Understanding the Brain Body Association

At its center, the psyche body association envelops the bidirectional correspondence between the cerebrum and body, interceded by a perplexing organization of brain hormonal, and biochemical pathways. The mind frequently viewed as the seat of cognizance and discernment, applies a significant effect on physical processes, for example, pulse, circulatory strain, insusceptible capability, and chemical emission. Alternately, physiological cycles inside the body can impact mental and close to home states deeply shaping contemplations, sentiments, and ways of behaving.

# Neurological Systems

Neuroscience research has clarified the brain components fundamental the psyche body association, featuring the job of the focal and fringe sensory systems in interceding the communication among mental and actual cycles. The autonomic sensory system, contained the thoughtful and parasympathetic branches, assumes a key part in controlling physiological reactions to stress, feelings, and natural boosts. Initiation of the thoughtful sensory system sets off the "instinctive" reaction, assembling the body's assets to adapt to apparent dangers, while actuation of the parasympathetic sensory system advances unwinding and supportive cycles.

# Hormonal Pathways

Chemicals, compound couriers discharged by different organs all through the body, likewise assume a vital part in the brain body association. The hypothalamic-pituitary-adrenal (HPA) pivot, for instance, manages the body's reaction to stretch by delivering cortisol and other pressure chemicals because of seen dangers or difficulties. Constant pressure can deregulate the HPA pivot, prompting raised cortisol levels and expanded chance of medical issues like nervousness, sorrow, cardiovascular infection, and resistant brokenness.

# Profound and Mental Elements

Feelings and mental states like pressure, tension, wretchedness, and flexibility apply a significant effect on actual wellbeing and prosperity. Constant pressure, described by diligent initiation of the body's pressure reaction frameworks, can add to an extensive variety of medical issues, including hypertension, diabetes, corpulence, and immune system problems. Then again, positive feelings like satisfaction, appreciation, and love have been related with worked on resistant capability, cardiovascular wellbeing, and life span.

# Psychoneuroimmunology

Psychoneuroimmunology (PNI) is a field of examination that investigates the communications between the apprehensive, endocrine, and safe frameworks underscoring the job of mental and profound variables in regulating resistant capability and illness powerlessness. Concentrates in PNI have exhibited the effect of pressure, social confinement, and pessimistic feelings on resistant capability, irritation, and powerlessness to irresistible and immune system sicknesses. On the other hand, mediations like care contemplation, unwinding strategies, and social help have been displayed to upgrade resistant capability, lessen aggravation, and further develop wellbeing results.

# The Job of Care and Contemplation

Care, the act of nonjudgmental consciousness of present second insight, has arisen as an amazing asset for developing the brain body association and advancing wellbeing and prosperity. Care contemplation includes deliberately focusing on tangible encounters like the breath, body sensations, considerations, and feelings, without connection or revulsion. By developing care, people can foster more noteworthy consciousness of their viewpoints, feelings, and substantial sensations, advancing pressure decrease, close to home guideline, and flexibility.

## Psychosocial Variables

Psychosocial factors like social help, financial status, and natural impacts additionally assume a huge part in shaping the brain body association. Social help, characterized as the discernment or experience of being really focused on, esteemed, and regarded by others, has been displayed to support against the adverse consequences of stress, advance flexibility, and improve physical and emotional well-being. Then again, social separation, forlornness, and saw social dismissal have been related with expanded hazard of sadness, tension, cardiovascular illness, and mortality.

# Integrative Medication Approaches

Integrative medication approaches like needle therapy, yoga, jujitsu, and qigong offer comprehensive strategies for advancing wellbeing and prosperity by tending to the brain body association. Needle therapy, a conventional Chinese medication work on including the inclusion of slender needles into explicit focuses on the body, has been displayed to tweak the autonomic sensory system, diminish irritation, and reduce torment. Yoga, a psyche body practice that joins actual stances, breath control, and reflection, has been related with further developed adaptability, strength, balance, and close to home prosperity.

## Functional Applications

Integrating mind-body rehearses into day to day existence can upgrade the brain body association and advance wellbeing and prosperity. A few useful applications include:

## *Care Reflection:*

Put away opportunity every day for care contemplation work on, zeroing in on developing present-second mindfulness and nonjudgmental acknowledgment of considerations, feelings, and sensations.

## *Yoga and Jujitsu:*

Go to yoga or jujitsu classes routinely to further develop adaptability, strength, equilibrium, and unwinding. Pick classes that stress care, breathe mindfulness, and delicate development to advance the brain body association.

## *Social Help:*

Develop significant associations with companions, family, and local area individuals to advance social help, association, and having a place. Connect for help during seasons of pressure or trouble, and proposition backing to others out of luck.

# End

All in all, the brain body association addresses a significant and multifaceted transaction among mental and actual wellbeing, with broad ramifications for by and large prosperity. By getting it and sustaining this association through practices like care contemplation, yoga, social help, and integrative medication draws near, people can upgrade their strength, decrease pressure, and advance wellbeing and essentialness. By developing more noteworthy consciousness of the brain body association and its effect on wellbeing, we can enable ourselves to live more adjusted, satisfying lives, with amicability and reconciliation between psyche, body, and soul.

# Chapter 6
# Flexibility and Joint Health

Adaptability and joint wellbeing are complicatedly connected parts of actual prosperity that assume urgent parts in keeping up with portability, capability, and generally personal satisfaction. Adaptability alludes to the capacity of muscles and connective tissues to protract and travel through a full scope of movement, while joint wellbeing envelops the state of the joints, including their construction, capability, and uprightness. In this complete investigation, we dive into the connection among adaptability and joint wellbeing, looking at the elements that impact both and investigating methodologies for advancing adaptability, forestalling injury, and safeguarding joint capability all through the life expectancy.

# Grasping Adaptability and Joint Wellbeing

Adaptability is fundamental for keeping up with ideal joint capability, as it takes into consideration smooth, unhindered development and forestalls firmness, agony, and injury. Tight muscles and connective tissues can limit joint portability, prompting compensatory development designs, expanded weight on the joints, and a higher gamble of injury. Alternately, keeping up with adaptability through customary extending and versatility activities can work on joint portability, decrease muscle pressure, and improve by and large actual execution.

Joint wellbeing envelops different variables, including the design and respectability of the joints, the soundness of encompassing muscles and connective tissues, and the presence of irritation, degeneration, or injury. Sound joints are portrayed by smooth, torment free development, satisfactory grease and padding, and ideal arrangement and dependability. Factors like age, hereditary qualities, way of life, and movement level can impact joint wellbeing, with specific circumstances like joint inflammation, osteoporosis, and injury presenting dangers to joint honesty and capability.

# Advantages of Adaptability for Joint Wellbeing

Adaptability assumes a significant part in advancing joint wellbeing and forestalling outer muscle issues like solidness, torment, and brokenness. A portion of the critical advantages of adaptability for joint wellbeing include:

# *Further developed Scope of Movement:*

Adaptability practices help keep up with or increment joint versatility, considering a more prominent scope of movement and improving adaptability in muscles and connective tissues encompassing the joint. Further developed scope of movement can decrease solidness, upgrade joint grease, and advance smooth, torment free development.

## Diminished Hazard of Injury:

Keeping up with ideal adaptability can assist with forestalling wounds by diminishing the gamble of muscle strains, tendon injuries, and joint separations. Adaptable muscles and connective tissues are better ready to assimilate and disperse powers during development, diminishing the stress on the joints and diminishing the probability of injury.

## Upgraded Joint Dependability:

Adaptability activities can work on joint soundness by advancing ideal arrangement, equilibrium, and coordination. Reinforcing and extending muscles encompassing the joint can help support and balance out the joint, lessening the gamble of flimsiness, misalignment, and injury.

## Easing of Joint Torment:

Adaptability activities can assist with mitigating joint torment by diminishing muscle strain, further developing flow, and advancing unwinding. Extending tight muscles and connective tissues can assuage strain on the joints, lighten solidness, and lessen irritation, prompting diminished torment and uneasiness.

# *Deferral of Joint Degeneration:*

Keeping up with adaptability and joint versatility can assist with postponing the beginning of joint degeneration and age-related changes like osteoarthritis. By advancing joint wellbeing and capability, adaptability activities can assist with protecting joint honesty and portability, empowering people to keep a functioning and autonomous way of life as they age.

Factors Affecting Adaptability and Joint Wellbeing
A few elements impact adaptability and joint wellbeing, including:

# *Age:*

Adaptability will in general diminish with age because of changes in muscle versatility, joint grease, and connective tissue adaptability. Maturing can likewise build the gamble of joint degeneration and conditions, for example, joint inflammation, which can influence joint wellbeing and capability.

# *Genetics:*

Hereditary qualities assume a part in deciding individual contrasts in adaptability and joint wellbeing. Certain individuals might be normally more adaptable or have an inclination to specific joint circumstances in light of hereditary variables.

## *Active work:*

Standard actual work, including extending, portability activities, and strength preparing, can advance adaptability and joint wellbeing by further developing muscle strength, adaptability, and joint solidness. In any case, unnecessary or ill-advised exercise can expand the gamble of injury and joint mileage.

## *Injury and Injury:*

Wounds like injuries, strains, and breaks can influence joint wellbeing by making harm the encompassing muscles, tendons, and ligament. Legitimate recovery and injury counteraction methodologies are fundamental for keeping up with joint trustworthiness and capability.

## *Stance and Arrangement:*

Unfortunate stance and arrangement can add to joint solidness, agony, and brokenness by putting unjustifiable weight on the joints and encompassing designs. Revising stance awkward nature and keeping up with appropriate arrangement during development are fundamental for safeguarding joint wellbeing.

Methodologies for Advancing Adaptability and Joint Wellbeing
To advance adaptability and joint wellbeing, consider integrating the accompanying methodologies into your everyday daily schedule:

## *Extending Activities:*

 Incorporate standard extending practices in your wellness routine to further develop adaptability and joint portability. Center on extending all significant muscle gatherings, including those encompassing the joints, and hold each stretch for 15-30 seconds to accomplish ideal outcomes.

## *Versatility Work:*

Consolidate versatility activities, for example, joint turns, dynamic stretches, and froth moving to work on joint portability and lessen firmness. Perform portability practices consistently, particularly when exercises, to set up the joints for development and forestall injury.

## *Strength Preparing:*

 Incorporate strength preparing practices in your gym routine daily schedule to develop muscle fortitude and soundness around the joints. Reinforcing the muscles encompassing the joints can help support and safeguard the joints, diminishing the gamble of injury and working on joint capability.

## *Legitimate Arrangement:*

 Focus on your stance and arrangement during day to day exercises and exercise. Pursue great stance routines like sitting and standing tall, keeping the spine unbiased, and staying away from over the top weight on the joints.

## Joint-Accommodating Exercises:

Pick low-effect  and joint-accommodating exercises like swimming, cycling, and yoga to diminish weight on the joints and limit the gamble of injury. Stay away from high-influence exercises or redundant developments that can compound joint agony and irritation.

## Sustenance and Hydration:

Keep a decent eating routine plentiful in supplements like nutrients, minerals, cell reinforcements, and omega-3 unsaturated fats, which backing joint wellbeing and decrease irritation. Remain hydrated by drinking a satisfactory measure of water every day to keep joints greased up and working ideally.

## Rest and Recuperation:

Permit your body time to rest and recuperate between exercises to forestall abuse wounds and advance joint wellbeing. Integrate rest days into your preparation plan and pay attention to your body's signs of exhaustion or uneasiness.

# End

Taking everything into account, adaptability and joint wellbeing are fundamental parts of generally actual prosperity, with significant ramifications for portability, capability, and personal satisfaction. By understanding the connection among adaptability and joint wellbeing and integrating procedures to advance both, people can decrease the gamble of injury, mitigate joint agony, and safeguard joint capability all through the life expectancy. Whether through extending, versatility works out, strength preparing, or way of life adjustments, putting resources into adaptability and joint wellbeing is an interest in long haul actual wellbeing and essentialness.

# Chapter 7
# Flexibility and Chronic Pain

Ongoing torment is a complicated and weakening condition that influences a great many individuals around the world, influencing actual capability, close to home prosperity, and personal satisfaction. While ongoing torment can emerge from different hidden causes, like injury, disease, or neurological brokenness, it frequently includes a critical part of muscle strain, solidness, and diminished adaptability. In this complete investigation, we dive into the complex connection among adaptability and persistent agony, analyzing how disabled adaptability can add to torment side effects and investigating remedial methodologies for overseeing ongoing agony through adaptability upgrading mediations.

## Figuring out Ongoing Torment

Constant torment is characterized as diligent agony going on for a considerable length of time or longer, past the typical time for tissue recuperating. Not at all like intense torment, which fills in as an advance notice sign of tissue harm or injury, ongoing torment can endure long after the underlying injury has recuperated and might not have an unmistakable physiological reason. Ongoing torment can appear in different structures, including outer muscle torment, neuropathic torment, fibromyalgia, and constant cerebral pain problems, and can altogether affect physical, close to home, and social working.

# The Job of Adaptability in Constant Agony

Adaptability assumes a vital part in the experience of constant torment, as close muscles and connective tissues can add to torment side effects by overburdening joints, packing nerves, and confining development. Weakened adaptability can prompt muscle irregular characteristics, unfortunate stance, adjusted development designs, and expanded hazard of injury, all of which can intensify persistent agony side effects. Moreover, constant torment itself can add to muscle strain and firmness, making an endless loop of agony and diminished adaptability.

# Normal Ongoing Torment Conditions

A few ongoing aggravation conditions are related with weakened adaptability and muscle strain, including:

## *Low Back Torment:*

Snugness in the muscles of the lower back, hips, and hamstrings is a typical contributing component to low back torment. Diminished adaptability in these muscle gatherings can prompt unfortunate stance, spinal misalignment, and expanded weight on the lumbar spine adding to agony and distress.

## *Neck and Shoulder Torment:*

Constant pressure and solidness in the muscles of the neck, shoulders, and upper back can prompt neck torment, migraines, and shoulder impingement condition. Unfortunate stance, delayed sitting, and dreary developments can compound muscle snugness and add to ongoing agony around there.

## *Fibromyalgia:*

Fibromyalgia is a persistent aggravation condition described by boundless outer muscle torment, exhaustion, and delicate focuses all through the body. Muscle firmness, decreased adaptability, and hyperalgesia (expanded aversion to torment) are normal highlights of fibromyalgia, adding to the general aggravation experience.

## *Arthritis:*

Joint pain, a gathering of fiery joint illnesses, can prompt persistent torment, solidness, and diminished scope of movement in impacted joints. Muscle snugness and shortcoming encompassing ligament joints can additionally restrict portability and fuel torment side effects.

Helpful Methodologies for Overseeing Ongoing Agony through Adaptability

Tending to adaptability deficiencies and muscle strain is a fundamental part of thorough agony the board methodologies for persistent agony. A few restorative methodologies can assist with further developing adaptability, diminish muscle strain, and reduce torment side effects:

## Extending Activities:

Integrate customary extending practices into your everyday daily schedule to further develop adaptability, diminish muscle pressure, and reduce torment side effects. Center around  extending tight muscles and connective tissues encompassing the impacted regions, for example, the lower back, neck, shoulders, and hips.

## Yoga and Pilates:

Partake in yoga or Pilates classes, which join extending, reinforcing, and care methods to advance adaptability, further develop act, and lessen pressure. These psyche body practices can assist with easing ongoing agony by addressing both physical and profound elements adding to torment side effects.

## Manual Treatment:

Search out the administrations of a certified manual specialist, like an actual specialist, alignment specialist, or back rub advisor, who can give involved methods to deliver muscle pressure, work on joint portability, and decrease torment. Modalities, for example, Myofascial discharge, trigger point treatment, and joint assembly can target explicit areas of strain and brokenness.

## Froth Rolling and Self-Myofascial Delivery:

Utilize a froth roller or self-knead devices to perform self-Myofascial discharge procedures, which can assist with delivering muscle pressure, further develop course, and upgrade adaptability. Center around carrying out close or delicate region of the body, applying delicate strain to deliver attachments and trigger focuses.

## Care Based Pressure Decrease:

Partake in care based pressure decrease (MBSR) programs, which show care reflection, delicate development, and unwinding strategies to diminish pressure, upgrade mindfulness, and further develop adapting abilities. Care practices can assist people with overseeing constant torment all the more successfully by developing acknowledgment, flexibility, and close to home prosperity.

## Amphibian Treatment:

Consider taking part in oceanic treatment or hydrotherapy programs, which include practices and stretches acted in a warm water pool. The lightness and opposition of water can offer delicate help and obstruction, making it more straightforward to move and stretch without putting unreasonable weight on the joints.

## *Slow Activity Movement:*

Steadily progress practice power and length to abstain from fueling torment side effects or causing injury. Begin with delicate, low-influence exercises like strolling, swimming, or cycling, and progressively increment power and term as endured. Pay attention to your body's signs and adjust practices on a case by case basis to keep away from overexertion.

# End

All in all, adaptability shortfalls and muscle strain assume critical parts in the experience of persistent agony, adding to torment side effects, utilitarian constraints, and decreased personal satisfaction. Tending to adaptability and versatility issues through restorative mediations like extending works out, yoga, manual treatment, and care based practices can assist with mitigating torment, work on actual capability, and improve in general prosperity for people living with persistent agony conditions. By integrating adaptability upgrading methodologies into complete agony the executives plans, people can enable themselves to play a functioning job in dealing with their aggravation and recovering their wellbeing and essentialness.

# Chapter 8
# Flexibility and Injury Prevention

Wounds are an awful reality for some people, whether they happen during sports, exercise, or day to day exercises. While a wounds are inescapable because of mishaps or outer variables, many can be forestalled through proactive measures, for example, adaptability preparing. Adaptability, the capacity of muscles and connective tissues to protract and travel through a full scope of movement, assumes a vital part in physical issue counteraction by upgrading joint portability, further developing development mechanics, and lessening the gamble of muscle strains, tendon injuries, and other normal wounds. In this far reaching investigation, we dig into the complex connection among adaptability and injury counteraction, analyzing the advantages of adaptability for decreasing injury risk and investigating methodologies for integrating adaptability preparing into your wellness schedule.

Figuring out the Job of Adaptability in Injury Counteraction Adaptability is a vital part of actual wellness that is much of the time neglected in injury counteraction programs. Notwithstanding, keeping up with ideal adaptability is fundamental for decreasing the gamble of injury and advancing protected and powerful development. Adaptability permits muscles and connective tissues to stretch and travel through their full scope of movement, which is basic for legitimate joint capability, biomechanics and development effectiveness. Without sufficient adaptability, muscles and connective tissues can turn out to be tight and limited, prompting compensatory development designs, adjusted biomechanics, and expanded hazard of injury.

# Advantages of Adaptability for Injury Anticipation

Adaptability preparing offers various advantages for injury anticipation, including:

## *Worked on Joint Versatility:*

Adaptability practices help keep up with or increment joint versatility, considering smooth and unhindered development. Further developed joint versatility diminishes the gamble of joint solidness, compensatory development examples, and abuse wounds by guaranteeing that joints can move unreservedly through their full scope of movement.

## *Improved Development Mechanics:*

Ideal adaptability is fundamental for legitimate development mechanics and biomechanics. By further developing adaptability in muscles and connective tissues encompassing the joints, people can perform developments with more prominent effectiveness, soundness, and control, diminishing the gamble of unfortunate method, flawed development examples, and injury.

## Decreased Muscle Strain and Firmness:

Adaptability preparing diminishes muscle pressure and solidness, which are normal antecedents to muscle strains and other delicate tissue wounds. By advancing unwinding and extension of muscles and connective tissues, adaptability activities can mitigate muscle snugness, further develop dissemination, and diminish the gamble of injury.

## Anticipation of Muscle Lopsided characteristics:

Adaptability preparing can assist with forestalling muscle lopsided characteristics by guaranteeing that contradicting muscle bunches have comparative adaptability and length pressure connections. Muscle uneven characters, where one muscle bunch is more tight or more fragile than its contradicting partner, can prompt modified joint mechanics, expanded weight on joints, and a raised gamble of injury.

## Easing of Abuse Wounds:

Abuse wounds, like tendinitis, bursitis, and stress cracks, can result from dull developments or over the top burden on muscles and connective tissues. Adaptability preparing lessens the gamble of abuse wounds by further developing tissue versatility, expanding strength to dreary pressure, and advancing tissue recuperation and fix.

## Integrating Adaptability Preparing into Your Wellness Schedule

To receive the rewards of adaptability for injury anticipation, consider integrating the accompanying methodologies into your wellness schedule:

## *Dynamic Warm-Up:*

Start every exercise with a unique warm-up that incorporates dynamic extending activities to set up your muscles and joints for development. Dynamic stretches include moving the body through a full scope of movement in a controlled way, assisting with expanding blood stream, further develop adaptability, and upgrade neuromuscular enactment.

## *Static Extending:*

Incorporate static extending practices toward the finish of your exercise or as a component of a cool-down daily schedule to further develop adaptability and advance unwinding. Center around extending all significant muscle gatherings, holding each stretch for 15-30 seconds to accomplish ideal outcomes. Static extending prolongs muscles and connective tissues, decrease muscle pressure and work on joint versatility.

## Froth Rolling and Self-Myofascial Delivery:

Utilize a froth roller or self-rub instruments to perform self-Myofascial discharge methods, focusing on close or delicate region of the body. Froth moving assists discharge with muscling pressure, ease trigger focuses, and further develop tissue versatility, upgrading adaptability and decreasing the gamble of injury. Center around carrying out significant muscle gatherings like the calves, hamstrings, quadriceps, and back.

## Yoga and Pilates:

Integrate yoga or Pilate's classes into your wellness routine to further develop adaptability, equilibrium, and center strength. Both yoga and Pilates accentuate adaptability, portability, and body mindfulness, making them powerful apparatuses for injury counteraction. Pick classes that attention on delicate extending, controlled development, and appropriate arrangement to limit the gamble of injury.

## Versatility Work:

Perform portability practices that target explicit joints and development examples to work on joint versatility and lessen solidness. Incorporate activities, for example, joint revolutions, dynamic stretches, and portability drills to address areas of snugness or limitation and further develop generally development quality.

## *Slow Movement:*

Slowly progress the power and span of your adaptability preparing to try not to overextend or causing injury. Begin with delicate stretches and steadily increment the force, term, and recurrence of your adaptability practices as your adaptability improves and your body adjusts to the requests of preparing.

Normal Adaptability Preparing Slip-ups to Keep away from While adaptability preparing offers various advantages for injury anticipation, it's vital for approach it with alert and keep away from normal slip-ups that can expand the gamble of injury:

## *Overstretching:*

Try not to overextend or constraining your body into positions past its ongoing scope of movement. Overextending can prompt muscle strains, tendon injuries, and joint unsteadiness, expanding the gamble of injury instead of forestalling it.

## *Bobbing or Snapping Developments:*

Abstain from bobbing or snapping developments during extending works out, as this can cause micro trauma to muscles and connective tissues, prompting injury. All things considered, perform static stretches with smooth, controlled developments and spotlight on bit by bit protracting the muscles without causing distress or torment.

## *Overlooking Muscle Uneven characters:*

Address muscle irregular characteristics through designated extending and reinforcing activities to forestall compensatory development designs and decrease the gamble of injury. Focus on areas of snugness or shortcoming and consolidate practices that focus on these areas to advance equilibrium and evenness in the body.

## *Skirting Warm-Up or Chill Off:*

Continuously start your exercise with a dynamic get ready to set up your muscles and joints for development and diminish the gamble of injury. In like manner, incorporate static extending practices toward the finish of your exercise or as a feature of a cool-down daily schedule to advance unwinding, adaptability, and muscle recuperation.

## *Disregarding Recuperation:*

Permit your body time to recuperate between adaptability instructional meetings to forestall abuse wounds and advance tissue fix and transformation. Integrate rest days into your preparation plan and pay attention to your body's signs to keep away from overtraining or pushing through torment.

# End

All in all, adaptability preparing is an important device for injury counteraction, assisting with working on joint versatility, improve development mechanics, and diminish the gamble of muscle strains, tendon injuries, and other normal wounds. By integrating adaptability practices into your wellness routine and tending to muscle irregular characteristics and development limitations, you can upgrade your body's strength to injury and work on generally actual execution. Whether through powerful extending, static extending, froth rolling, or versatility drills, putting resources into adaptability is an interest in sans injury and effective development for a better, more dynamic way of life.

# Chapter 9
# Incorporating Flexibility into Daily Life

Adaptability is a key part of actual wellness that frequently assumes a lower priority in our bustling lives. Nonetheless, keeping up with ideal adaptability is fundamental for generally wellbeing and prosperity, as it advances joint versatility, diminishes muscle strain, further develops stance, and improves development effectiveness. While committed adaptability instructional meetings are gainful, coordinating adaptability practices into your day to day schedule can assist you with receiving the rewards of expanded adaptability and advance long haul wellbeing and imperativeness. In this exhaustive investigation, we dig into commonsense procedures for integrating adaptability into day to day existence, offering tips and strategies for further developing adaptability and upgrading generally speaking actual prosperity.

## Grasping the Significance of Adaptability

Adaptability alludes to the capacity of muscles and connective tissues to extend and travel through a full scope of movement. Ideal adaptability is fundamental for keeping up with joint portability, lessening the gamble of injury, and advancing productive development designs.

Tight muscles and connective tissues can confine joint versatility, increment the gamble of muscle strains and tendon injuries, and add to unfortunate stance and development mechanics. By integrating adaptability practices into your day to day daily schedule, you can further develop adaptability, lessen muscle pressure, and upgrade by and large actual capability.

## Viable Procedures for Integrating Adaptability into Day to day existence

### *Early daytime Extending Schedule:*

Begin your day with a concise extending routine to awaken your muscles, slacken firm joints, and set up your body for the day ahead. Endure 5-10 minutes performing dynamic stretches, for example, arm circles, leg swings, and middle turns to increment blood stream, further develop adaptability, and stimulate your body and psyche.

### *Stretch Breaks at Work:*

Enjoy short stretch reprieves over the course of the day to battle the impacts of delayed sitting and lessen muscle pressure and firmness. Set a clock to remind yourself to stand up, stretch, and move around each hour or somewhere in the vicinity. Center around extending tight muscles like the neck, shoulders, hips, and lower back to mitigate pressure and further develop act.

## *Integrate Extending into Everyday Exercises:*

Search for valuable chances to integrate extending into everyday exercises like sitting in front of the television perusing, or holding up in line. Utilize business breaks or free time to perform basic stretches, for example, toe contacts, shoulder rolls, or calf stretches to keep your muscles nimble and adaptable.

## *Work area Stretches:*

Perform work area stretches to reduce muscle pressure and further develop pose during extended periods of time of sitting at work or examining. Stretch your neck, shoulders, chest, and back by performing situated stretches, for example, neck slants, shoulder rolls, chest openers, and situated spinal turns. Hold each stretch for 15-30 seconds and rehash a few times over the course of the day.

## *Evening Extending Schedule:*

Wind down by the day's end with a loosening up night extending routine to deliver strain, advance unwinding, and set up your body for supportive rest. Zero in on delicate stretches that target tight muscles and advance unwinding, like forward twists, hip openers, and spinal turns. Consolidate profound breathing and care strategies to upgrade the unwinding reaction and advance peaceful rest.

## Yoga or Pilates Practice:

Integrate yoga or Pilates into your week after week schedule to further develop adaptability, strength, and body mindfulness. Go to yoga or Pilates classes at a nearby studio or follow online recordings and instructional exercises to rehearse at home. Pick classes that emphasis on adaptability, versatility, and unwinding to receive the most extreme rewards for your body and brain.

## Froth Rolling:

Utilize a froth roller or self-rub devices to perform self-Myofascial discharge methods to deliver muscle strain and further develop adaptability. Burn through 5-10 minutes froth moving tight or delicate region of the body like the calves, hamstrings, quadriceps, gluts, and back Apply delicate tenslon and roll gradually over each muscle gathering to deliver bonds and trigger focuses.

## Dynamic Way of life Decisions:

Settle on dynamic way of life decisions that advance adaptability and development over the course of the day. Use the stairwell rather than the lift, walk or bicycle to work, and integrate actual work into your everyday schedule whenever the situation allows. Participate in exercises that advance adaptability, like swimming moving, or climbing, to keep your body agile and versatile.

# Advantages of Integrating Adaptability into Day to day existence

Integrating adaptability into your day to day routine offers various advantages for physical, mental, and profound prosperity, including:

## *Worked on Joint Portability:*

 Normal adaptability practices help keep up with or increment joint portability, taking into account smooth and unhindered development. Further developed joint versatility lessens the gamble of joint firmness, upgrades development proficiency, and advances better generally speaking actual capability.

## *Diminished Muscle Pressure and Firmness:*

Extending and adaptability practices assist with lessening muscle strain and firmness, easing distress and advancing unwinding. By delivering pressure in close muscles and connective tissues, adaptability activities can assist with diminishing pressure, further develop flow, and upgrade sensations of prosperity.

## *Upgraded Stance and Arrangement:*

Preparing advances  legitimate stance and arrangement by protracting tight muscles and revising strong irregular characteristics. Further developed act decreases the gamble of outer muscle torment and brokenness, upgrades breathing and course, and advances by and large spinal wellbeing.

## *Injury Avoidance:*

Keeping up with ideal adaptability diminishes the gamble of muscle strains, tendon injuries, and other normal wounds by working on joint versatility and development mechanics. By integrating adaptability practices into your day to day daily schedule, you can diminish the gamble of injury and remain dynamic and sans injury.

## *Stress Alleviation and Unwinding:*

Adaptability practices advance unwinding and stress alleviation by enacting the body's unwinding reaction and advancing the arrival of endorphins, the body's normal pain relievers. By integrating extending and unwinding strategies into your everyday daily practice, you can diminish pressure, further develop state of mind, and improve generally speaking personal satisfaction.

# Tips for Progress

To expand the advantages of integrating adaptability into your day to day routine, think about the accompanying tips:

Begin gradually and step by step increment the power and length of your adaptability practices after some time.

Pay attention to your body and try not to propel yourself past your cutoff points. Stretch to the mark of gentle distress, not torment.

Remain steady and focus on adaptability in your day to day everyday practice. Put away  opportunity every day for extending and unwinding works out.

Be aware of legitimate method and arrangement during extending activities to keep away from injury and expand viability.

Explore different avenues regarding various sorts of adaptability activities to find what turns out best for your body and inclinations.

Remain hydrated and fed to help your body's recuperation and transformation to adaptability preparing.

Integrate care procedures, for example, profound breathing and perception to improve the unwinding reaction and advance more prominent psyche body mindfulness.

# End

All in all, integrating adaptability into your regular routine is fundamental for advancing ideal physical, mental, and closes to home prosperity. By coordinating adaptability practices into your day to day daily schedule, you can work on joint versatility, decrease muscle strain, improve stance and arrangement, forestall wounds and advance unwinding and stress help. Whether through morning extends, work area extends, yoga classes, or froth moving meetings, tracking down ways of integrating adaptability into your everyday existence can significantly affect your general wellbeing and essentialness. Focus on focusing on adaptability, and receive the benefits of a more adaptable tough, and dynamic body and brain.

# Chapter 10
# Nutrition for Flexibility and Pain Reduction

Nourishment assumes a central part in supporting by and large wellbeing and prosperity, including adaptability and torment decrease. While we frequently partner sustenance with weight the board or energy levels, the food varieties we eat likewise essentially affect aggravation, joint wellbeing, muscle capability, and recuperation from wounds. In this thorough investigation, we dive into the connection between nourishment, adaptability, and torment decrease, analyzing how dietary decisions can impact irritation, joint wellbeing, and outer muscle capability. We'll likewise investigate explicit supplements and dietary examples that help adaptability and agony decrease, engaging you to go with informed decisions to sustain your body and upgrade your general personal satisfaction.

## Figuring out the Job of Sustenance in Adaptability and Torment Decrease

Appropriate nourishment gives the fundamental supplements and energy our bodies need to ideally work.

With regards to adaptability and agony decrease sustenance assumes a few key parts:

## Lessening Irritation:

Ongoing irritation is a typical hidden consider numerous outer muscle conditions, including joint pain, tendonitis, and muscle strains. Certain food varieties and dietary examples can either advance or lessen irritation in the body, affecting agony levels and joint capability.

## Supporting Joint Wellbeing:

Supplements like collagen, omega-3 unsaturated fats, and cell reinforcements assume basic parts in supporting joint wellbeing, ligament uprightness, and oil. An eating routine wealthy in these supplements can assist with keeping up with joint portability, decrease solidness, and forestall degenerative changes related with maturing and persistent circumstances.

## Streamlining Muscle Capability:

Sufficient admission of protein, amino acids, and micronutrients is fundamental for muscle fix, recuperation, and capability. Legitimate sustenance upholds muscle development, strength, and adaptability, lessening the gamble of muscle strains and upgrading in general actual execution.

*Advancing Generally speaking Prosperity:*

Nourishment influences different parts of generally speaking wellbeing and prosperity, including energy levels state of mind, and mental capability. By feeding your body with supplement thick food varieties, you can uphold ideal physical and mental capability, lessening pressure and improving versatility to agony and inconvenience.

## Key Supplements for Adaptability and Torment Decrease

*Omega-3 Unsaturated fats:*

Omega-3 unsaturated fats tracked down in greasy fish, flaxseeds, chia seeds, and pecans, have calming properties that can assist with diminishing irritation and lighten joint agony. Integrating omega-3-rich food varieties into your eating regimen might assist with working on joint versatility and adaptability.

*Collagen:*

Collagen is the really underlying protein in connective tissues like ligaments, tendons, and ligament. Devouring collagen-rich food sources or enhancements might assist with supporting joint wellbeing, diminish joint agony, and further develop adaptability. Wellsprings of collagen incorporate bone stock, collagen enhancements, and gelatin-rich food sources like bone-in meats and poultry.

## Antioxidants:

Cancer prevention agents like nutrients C and E,
Beta-carotene, and polyphenols, assist with diminishing oxidative pressure and irritation in the body. Consuming different bright foods grown from the ground, as well as nuts, seeds, and entire grains, can give many cell reinforcements to help joint wellbeing and diminish torment.

## Protein:

Protein is fundamental for muscle fix, recuperation, and development. Consuming a satisfactory measure of top notch protein from sources like lean meats, poultry, fish, eggs, dairy items, vegetables, and tofu can uphold muscle capability and adaptability, lessening the gamble of muscle strains and wounds.

## Vitamin D:

Vitamin D assumes an urgent part in bone wellbeing and safe capability. Sufficient vitamin D levels might assist with lessening aggravation, work on joint capability, and mitigate outer muscle torment. Wellsprings of vitamin D incorporate daylight openness, greasy fish, braced dairy items, and vitamin D enhancements.

## *Magnesium:*

Magnesium is engaged with muscle unwinding, nerve capability, and bone wellbeing. Eating magnesium-rich food varieties like verdant green vegetables, nuts, seeds, vegetables, and entire grains can assist with diminishing muscle pressure, advance unwinding, and reduce torment related with muscle spasms and firmness.

# Dietary Examples for Adaptability and Agony Decrease

Notwithstanding individual supplements, certain dietary examples might advance adaptability and agony decrease:

## *Calming Diet:*

A calming diet centers on entire, negligibly handled food sources that assist with lessening aggravation in the body. Underscore organic products, vegetables, greasy fish, nuts, seeds, olive oil, and flavors, for example, turmeric and ginger while limiting handled food varieties, refined carbs, sweet refreshments, and exorbitant liquor consumption.

## *Mediterranean Eating routine:*

The Mediterranean eating routine, wealthy in organic products, vegetables, entire grains, vegetables, olive oil and greasy fish, is related with diminished irritation, further developed heart wellbeing, and lower hazard of ongoing illnesses. Integrating Mediterranean-style feasts into your eating regimen might assist with supporting joint wellbeing and diminish agony and aggravation.

## *Plant-Based Diet:*

A plant-based diet stresses natural products, vegetables, nuts, seeds, and entire grains while limiting or wiping out creature items. Plant-based counts calories are wealthy in cell reinforcements, fiber, and phytonutrients, which can assist with lessening irritation, support joint wellbeing, and advance in general prosperity.

## *Flexitarian Diet:*

A Flexitarian diet is transcendently plant-based however takes into consideration periodic utilization of meat and creature items. Flexitarian consumes less calories are adaptable and adjustable, making them reasonable for people looking to integrate more plant-based food sources into their eating regimen while as yet getting a charge out of infrequent creature items for assortment and equilibrium.

# Viable Ways to integrate Adaptability Steady Sustenance into Your Eating regimen

## *Eat a Decent Eating regimen:*

Center around eating different supplement thick food sources from all nutrition classes, including organic products, vegetables, entire grains, lean proteins, and sound fats, to guarantee you're getting the fundamental supplements your body needs for adaptability and agony decrease.

## *Focus on Omega-3-Rich Food varieties:*

Incorporate greasy fish like salmon, mackerel, and sardines in your eating regimen consistently to help your admission of omega-3 unsaturated fats. In the event that you're veggie lover or vegetarian, consolidate plant-based wellsprings of omega-3s like flaxseeds, chia seeds, hemp seeds, and pecans into your feasts.

## *Consolidate Collagen-Rich Food sources:*

Integrate collagen-rich food varieties like bone stock gelatin, and collagen supplements into your eating regimen to help joint wellbeing and adaptability. Consider adding collagen powder to smoothies, soups, or drinks for a simple and advantageous method for supporting your collagen consumption.

## *Pick Brilliant Foods grown from the ground:*

Expect to remember different vivid products of the soil for your feasts to expand your admission of cell reinforcements and phytonutrients. Pick dynamic, profoundly shaded produce, for example, berries, mixed greens, chime peppers, and yams to help joint wellbeing and decrease irritation.

## *Decide on Lean Protein Sources:*

Pick lean protein sources like poultry, fish, tofu, tempeh, vegetables, and low-fat dairy items to help muscle fix recuperation, and adaptability. Integrate protein-rich food varieties into every feast and nibble to guarantee you're meeting your day to day protein needs.

## Remain Hydrated:

Drink a lot of water over the course of the day to remain hydrated and support by and large wellbeing and prosperity. Legitimate hydration is fundamental for keeping up with joint grease, muscle capability, and tissue versatility, all of which add to adaptability and agony decrease.

## Limit Handled Food varieties and Added Sugars:

Limit your admission of handled food varieties, refined starches, sweet bites, and improved drinks, as these food varieties can add to aggravation, joint agony, and diminished adaptability. Center around entire insignificantly handled food sources to help ideal wellbeing and imperativeness.

# End

All in all, sustenance assumes a urgent part in supporting adaptability and torment decrease by giving the fundamental supplements our bodies need for ideal outer muscle capability, joint wellbeing, and irritation the executives. By focusing on supplement thick food sources, integrating key supplements like omega-3 unsaturated fats, collagen, cell reinforcements, and protein into your eating regimen, and following adaptability steady dietary examples, for example, the Mediterranean eating routine or plant-based diet, you can support your body and advance adaptability, versatility, and generally prosperity. Make sure to remain hydrated, limit handled food sources and added sugars, and focus on entire, insignificantly handled food varieties to help your excursion toward ideal adaptability and agony free living. With careful eating and informed food decisions, you can fuel your body for more noteworthy adaptability, strength, and essentialness, upgrading your general personal satisfaction for quite a long time into the future.

# Chapter 11
# Overcoming Challenges

Life is loaded with difficulties, snags, and misfortunes that can test our strength, assurance, and capacity to adjust. Whether we're confronting individual battles, proficient mishaps, or wellbeing related impediments, beating difficulties is a fundamental ability for progress and satisfaction in all everyday issues. In this extensive investigation, we dig into the idea of difficulties, analyzing their effect on our lives and prosperity, and investigating systems for defeating affliction, building versatility, and flourishing notwithstanding deterrents.

## Grasping the Idea of Difficulties

Challenges come in different structures and can emerge from various parts of our lives, including:

## *Individual Difficulties:*

Individual difficulties might incorporate relationship hardships, family clashes, monetary issues, or psychological well-being issues like nervousness or gloom. These difficulties can affect our profound prosperity confidence, and feeling of satisfaction.

## *Proficient Difficulties:*

Proficient difficulties might incorporate employment cutback, vocation advances, working environment clashes, or challenges in accomplishing balance between fun and serious activities. These difficulties can influence our expert development, work fulfillment, and generally speaking vocation direction.

## *Wellbeing Difficulties:*

Wellbeing difficulties might incorporate constant ailments wounds, handicaps, or way of life related medical problems like stoutness or habit. These difficulties can affect our actual wellbeing, close to home prosperity, and personal satisfaction.

No matter what their inclination, difficulties can bring out sensations of stress, tension, dissatisfaction, or gloom. In any case, challenges likewise present open doors for development, learning, and self-disclosure. By embracing difficulties as any open doors for individual and expert turn of events, we can develop versatility, strength, and cleverness in exploring life's highs and lows.

# Techniques for Conquering Difficulties

## *Develop a Development Outlook:*

Embrace a development outlook, accepting that difficulties are potential open doors for learning and development as opposed to impossible snags. Embrace mishaps as important opportunities for growth, center around arrangements as opposed to harping on issues, and view disappointments as venturing stones to progress.

## *Foster Flexibility:*

Develop flexibility, the capacity to return from difficulty and flourish even with difficulties. Fabricate versatility by reinforcing your adapting abilities, keeping an uplifting perspective, cultivating social associations, and rehearsing taking care of oneself exercises like activity, care, and unwinding methods.

## *Put forth Reasonable Objectives:*

Put forth reasonable and attainable objectives that line up with your qualities, needs, and capacities. Break bigger objectives into more modest, reasonable advances, and praise progress and achievements en route. Change your objectives depending on the situation in light of changing conditions or criticism.

## Look for Help:

 Connect for help from companions, relatives, coaches, or experts during testing times. Encircle yourself with a strong organization of individuals who can offer consolation, counsel, and commonsense help when required. Make sure to for help or look for proficient direction while confronting overpowering difficulties.

## Practice Self-Empathy:

Practice self-empathy, treating you with consideration, understanding, and acknowledgment during troublesome times. Be delicate with yourself, recognize your assets and constraints, and keep away from self-analysis or negative self-talk. Indulge yourself with a similar generosity and sympathy you would propose to a companion out of luck.

## Center around Arrangements:

Center around finding  commonsense arrangements and finding a way proactive ways to address difficulties instead of harping on issues or mishaps. Separate complex difficulties into reasonable errands, conceptualize possible arrangements, and make a definitive move to push ahead.

## Keep up with Point of view:

Keep up with viewpoint and continue testing circumstances in setting by perceiving that misfortunes and snags are impermanent and reasonable. Practice appreciation for the positive parts of your life, think about past victories and flexibility, and help yourself to remember your assets and capacities.

## Gain from Disappointment:

Embrace disappointment as a characteristic piece of the educational experience and a chance for development and improvement. Dissect what turned out badly, recognize illustrations learned, and use disappointment as inspiration to attempt once more with a restored feeling of assurance and flexibility.

## Remain Adaptable and Versatile:

Remain adaptable and versatile despite challenges perceiving that change is inescapable and transformation is fundamental for endurance and achievement. Be available to novel thoughts, points of view, and amazing open doors, and change your arrangements or approach on a case by case basis to conquer obstructions and accomplish your objectives.

## Practice Constancy:

Practice determination and constancy in seeking after your objectives and defeating difficulties, even despite mishaps or impediments. Remain focused on your vision, keep an inspirational perspective, and continue to push ahead earnestly and versatility.

# Defeating Explicit Kinds of Difficulties
# Defeating Individual Difficulties:

## *Focus on Taking care of one:*

Deal with your physical, close to home, and mental prosperity by focusing on taking care of oneself exercises like activity, unwinding, side interests, and social associations.

## *Look for Proficient Assistance:*

On the off chance that you're battling with emotional well-being issues or individual issues, make it a point to proficient assistance from a specialist, instructor, or care group.

## *Put down stopping points:*

Lay out clear limits with others to safeguard your time, energy, and profound prosperity. Figure out how to express no to solicitations or responsibilities that overpower or deplete you.

# Beating Proficient Difficulties:

## *Foster New Abilities:*

Remain versatile and constantly foster your abilities and information to remain serious in the work environment. Search out open doors for proficient turn of events, preparing, or schooling to upgrade your profession possibilities.

## *Organization and Construct Connections:*

Develop proficient connections and organization with partners, coaches, and industry contacts to extend your chances and encouraging group of people.
Investigate New Open doors: Be available to investigating new vocation ways, ventures, or potential open doors that line up with your inclinations, values, and objectives. Think about independent work, counseling, or business as elective profession ways.

# Beating Wellbeing Difficulties:

## *Focus on Wellbeing and Health:*

Focus on your wellbeing by embracing a fair eating regimen, standard work-out daily practice, and sound way of life propensities that help your physical and mental prosperity.

## *Heed Clinical Guidance:*

Heed clinical guidance and therapy plans recommended by medical care experts to oversee ongoing diseases wounds or ailments really.

## *Practice Self-Sympathy:*

Be caring and patient with yourself as you explore wellbeing challenges, perceiving that mending takes time and advance might be progressive. Center on what you have some control over and celebrate little triumphs en route.

# End

All in all, defeating difficulties is a fundamental ability for progress and satisfaction in all everyday issues. By taking on a development outlook, creating strength, laying out reasonable objectives, looking for help, rehearsing self-empathy, and remaining adaptable and versatile, we can explore life's high points and low points with boldness, assurance, and beauty. Whether confronting individual battles, proficient mishaps, or wellbeing related deterrents, recall that difficulties are open doors for development, learning, and self-disclosure. Embrace difficulties as venturing stones to progress, and use them as impetuses for individual and expert turn of events. With tirelessness, versatility, and an uplifting perspective, you can conquer any test that comes your direction and arise more grounded, smarter, and stronger than any time in recent memory.

# Chapter 12
# Flexibility for Specific Populations

Adaptability is a pivotal part of actual wellbeing and prosperity, paying little heed to progress in years, capacity or foundation. Notwithstanding, certain populaces might confront extraordinary difficulties or contemplations with regards to further developing adaptability and versatility In this complete investigation, we dig into the significance of adaptability for explicit populaces, looking at custom-made practices, contemplations, and methodologies for advancing adaptability and upgrading generally personal satisfaction across different socioeconomics.

## Grasping the Significance of Adaptability for Explicit Populaces

Adaptability assumes a fundamental part in keeping up with actual capability, portability, and freedom for people of any age and capacities. Be that as it may, explicit populaces might experience novel difficulties or contemplations connected with adaptability:

## *Kids and Youths:*

 Developing bodies go through massive changes in outer muscle advancement, adaptability, and coordinated movements during youth and puberty. Adaptability preparing during these early stages can assist with supporting sound development and advancement, further develop pose, and decrease the gamble of wounds related with sports and proactive tasks.

## More seasoned Grown-ups:

Maturing is related with normal decreases in adaptability joint versatility, and muscle flexibility, which can add to solidness, diminished scope of movement, and expanded chance of falls and wounds. Adaptability practices for more seasoned grown-ups are fundamental for keeping up with portability, protecting utilitarian freedom, and improving personal satisfaction as they age.

## Competitors and Dynamic People:

Competitors and people participated in customary active work require ideal adaptability to perform at their best, forestall wounds, and backing recuperation. Explicit adaptability practices custom fitted to the requests of their game or action can assist with further developing execution, diminish muscle irregular characteristics, and upgrade generally athletic execution.

## People with Incapacities:

Individuals with incapacities might confront versatility limitations, muscle snugness, or joint impediments because of their particular condition or disability. Adjusted adaptability activities and alterations are fundamental for advancing versatility, further developing scope of movement, and upgrading actual capability and cooperation in everyday exercises.

## *Pregnant Ladies:*

Pregnancy can prompt changes in pose, weight circulation, and joint laxity, which might affect adaptability and versatility. Protected and delicate adaptability practices custom-made to the necessities and solace level of pregnant ladies can assist with lightening uneasiness lessen muscle strain, and backing generally prosperity during pregnancy and post pregnancy recuperation.

# Custom-made Practices and Contemplations for Explicit Populaces
# Kids and Young people:

## *Consolidate Energetic Exercises:*

Draw in youngsters and teenagers for entertainment only and energetic exercises that advance adaptability, like yoga, dance, vaulting, or hand to hand fighting. Accentuate satisfaction and investigation of development instead of severe adherence to conventional extending schedules.

## *Support Dynamic Play:*

Empower dynamic play and support in different games and proactive tasks to advance by and large actual turn of events, coordination, and adaptability. Give open doors to unstructured play and unconstrained development to help regular engine expertise improvement.

## *Center around Appropriate Strategy:*

Show kids and teenagers legitimate extending procedures, underlining the significance of heating up muscles prior to extending and trying not to skip or yanking developments that can cause injury. Energize continuous movement and adaptability acquires over the long run.

## **More established Grown-ups:**

## *Begin Gradually and Progress Steadily:*

Start adaptability practices for more established Grown-ups with delicate, low-influence developments and stretches to heat up muscles and joints. Progress to additional difficult activities bit by bit, considering individual capacities, solace level, and any previous medical issue.

## *Underline Utilitarian Developments:*

 Center around  adaptability practices that imitate useful developments and exercises of day to day living, like coming to, bowing, turning, and hunching down. Integrate practices that target significant muscle gatherings and joints, including the spine, hips, shoulders, and lower legs.

## *Incorporate Equilibrium and Security Preparing:*

Coordinate equilibrium and steadiness preparing into adaptability schedules for more seasoned grown-ups to lessen the gamble of falls and improve generally versatility and autonomy. Incorporate activities like remaining on one leg, heel-to-toe strolling, and balance difficulties utilizing solidness balls or froth cushions.

## Competitors and Dynamic People:

## *Recognize Game Explicit Requirements:*

 Distinguish the particular adaptability prerequisites of the competitor's game or action and designer adaptability preparing likewise. For instance, gymnasts might require more prominent adaptability in the shoulders and hips, while sprinters might profit from further developed adaptability in the hamstrings and calves.

## Integrate Dynamic Extending:

Focus on powerful extending practices that include controlled, dull developments through a full scope of movement to set up the body for action and improve strong execution. Dynamic extending can assist with further developing adaptability, versatility, and neuromuscular coordination.

## Incorporate Recuperation Practices:

Coordinate adaptability practices into post-exercise or recuperation schedules to help muscle recuperation, decrease irritation, and forestall injury. Incorporate froth rolling, self-Myofascial discharge, and delicate extending to lighten muscle pressure and advance unwinding.

## People with Inabilities:

## Tailor Activities to Individual Necessities:

Adjust adaptability activities to oblige the particular necessities and capacities of people with handicaps. Consider factors like portability restrictions, joint soundness, muscle shortcoming, and tactile responsive qualities while planning adaptability programs.

## *Utilize Assistive Gadgets and Backing:*

Consolidate assistive gadgets, versatile hardware, or backing from guardians or specialists to work with protected and compelling cooperation in adaptability works out. Uses props like lashes, blocks, or seats to adjust extend and give solidness and backing depending on the situation.

## *Center around Scope of Movement:*

Underscore practices that attention on further developing scope of movement, joint versatility, and muscle adaptability in people with handicaps. Incorporate delicate stretches and developments that target tight or confined muscles and joints while limiting inconvenience or strain.

## **Pregnant Ladies:**

## *Pick Protected and Delicate Activities:*

Select adaptability practices that are protected and agreeable for pregnant ladies to perform all through pregnancy. Keep away from practices that include lying level on the back or profound contorting developments, especially in the later phases of pregnancy.

## Change on a case by case basis:

Alter adaptability activities to oblige the changing necessities and actual limits of pregnant ladies as their pregnancy advances. Empower alterations, for example, involving props for help, decreasing the power or span of stretches, or keeping away from practices that cause distress or strain.

## Center around Pelvic Floor Wellbeing:

Integrate practices that advance pelvic floor wellbeing and strength, like Keels, pelvic slants, and hip-opening stretches. Accentuate unwinding and breathing strategies to lessen strain and advance unwinding in the pelvic region.

## End

All in all, adaptability is fundamental for advancing actual wellbeing, versatility, and by and large prosperity across different populaces. By understanding the remarkable difficulties and contemplations looked by unambiguous populaces, we can fit adaptability practices and procedures to address individual issues and inclinations. Whether working with youngsters and youths, more seasoned grown-ups, competitors, people with handicaps, or pregnant ladies, it's fundamental to focus on wellbeing, inclusivity, and versatility in adaptability programming. By advancing adaptability and versatility for all, we can engage people to upgrade their personal satisfaction, accomplish their objectives, and flourish in each phase of life and capacity.

# Chapter 13
# Integrative Approaches to Pain Management

Torment is an intricate and diverse experience that can significantly affect physical, close to home, and mental prosperity. While customary clinical medicines, for example, prescription and medical procedure assume a vital part in overseeing torment, they may not necessarily give total help or address the fundamental reasons for torment. Integrative ways to deal with torment the board offer all-encompassing methodologies that join regular medication with correlative and elective treatments to advance recuperating, diminish torment, and work on generally speaking personal satisfaction. In this complete investigation, we dive into integrative ways to deal with torment the board, looking at the standards, practices, and proof based systems for tending to torment according to a comprehensive point of view.

## Grasping Torment and Its Effect

Torment is a complex tangible and profound experience that can result from different variables, including injury, sickness, irritation, or mental pressure. Intense torment fills in as a defensive component, flagging tissue harm or injury and provoking the body to make a move to advance mending. In any case, persistent agony, enduring longer than three to a half year, can debilitate affect actual capability, versatility, and personal satisfaction.

Ongoing agony is in many cases joined by mental and close to home side effects like nervousness, sadness, and rest aggravations, which can additionally worsen the view of torment and debilitate generally prosperity. Also, persistent agony can add to decreased personal satisfaction, social detachment, handicap, and expanded medical care use and expenses.

# Standards of Integrative Agony The board

Integrative agony the board approaches perceive torment as a multi-layered encounter that requires an exhaustive and comprehensive way to deal with treatment. Key standards of integrative agony the executives include:

## *Individualized Care:*

Perceiving that aggravation is novel to every person, integrative agony the executive's approaches focus on customized care custom-made to the particular necessities, inclinations, and objectives of the patient.

## *Multimodal Treatment:*

Integrative torment the board uses a mix of regular clinical medicines, reciprocal treatments, and way of life mediations to address torment from numerous points and advance complete recuperating.

## Tending to the Main drivers:

Integrative methodologies mean to distinguish and address the hidden reasons for torment, instead of exclusively zeroing in on side effect the executives. By focusing on the underlying drivers of agony, integrative treatments can advance long haul help and recuperating.

## Engaging Patients:

Integrative agony the executives enables patients to play a functioning job in their mending cycle by giving schooling, assets, and backing to assist them with settling on informed conclusions about their wellbeing and prosperity.

## Cooperative Consideration:

Integrative agony the board includes cooperation among medical services suppliers from various disciplines, including doctors, actual specialists, clinicians, nutritionists, and correlative advisors, to give extensive and facilitated care.

# Proof Based Integrative Ways to deal with Agony the executives

## *Mind-Body Treatments:*

Mind-body treatments like care contemplation, yoga, judo, and qigong have been displayed to decrease torment, work on actual capability, and improve personal satisfaction in people with constant agony. These practices advance unwinding, stress decrease, and body mindfulness, assisting individuals with better adapting to agony and uneasiness.

## *Acupuncture:*

Needle therapy, an old Chinese treatment including the addition of meager needles into explicit focuses on the body, has been displayed to ease torment and advance mending in different persistent agony conditions, including back torment, osteoarthritis, and headaches. Needle therapy might work by animating the arrival of endorphins, serotonin, and different synapses that adjust torment insight and advance mending.

## *Manual Treatments:*

Manual treatments like chiropractic control, knead treatment, and osteopathic control can assist with lessening torment, work on joint versatility, and ease muscle pressure and solidness. These treatments center on reestablishing legitimate arrangement, decreasing irritation, and elevating dissemination to work with mending and relief from discomfort.

## Nourishing Treatment:

Sustenance assumes a vital part in irritation, torment discernment, and by and large wellbeing and prosperity. Integrative ways to deal with torment the executives might incorporate dietary mediations like calming consumes less calories, supplementation with supplements and botanicals with pain relieving properties, and customized sustenance intends to address explicit nourishing lacks and backing recuperating.

## Practice Treatment:

Ordinary active work and exercise have been displayed to lessen torment, work on actual capability, and upgrade mind-set and prosperity in people with constant agony conditions. Integrative agony the executive's projects might incorporate directed practice programs, non-intrusive treatment, and recovery practices custom-made to the singular's necessities and capacities.

## Mental Conduct Treatment (CBT):

Mental conduct treatment (CBT) is a psychotherapeutic methodology that helps people distinguish and change maladaptive considerations, convictions, and ways of behaving that add to agony and languishing. CBT strategies, for example, unwinding preparing, mental rebuilding, and stress the executives can assist people with creating adapting abilities, diminish torment power, and work on in general personal satisfaction.

## *Biofeedback:*

Biofeedback is a brain body strategy that assists people with figuring out how to control physiological cycles, for example, pulse, muscle strain, and skin temperature through visual or hear-able input. Biofeedback preparing can assist people with creating self-guideline abilities, decrease torment discernment, and advance unwinding and stress decrease.

## Incorporating Care into Torment the board

Care, the act of focusing on the current second with transparency, interest, and acknowledgment, is a center part of numerous integrative aggravations the executive's draws near. Care based mediations, for example, care reflection, body filter, and careful development have been displayed to lessen torment power, further develop torment related results, and upgrade in general prosperity in people with ongoing agony conditions.

Care rehearses advance consciousness of substantial sensations, feelings, and considerations connected with torment without judgment or opposition, assisting people with fostering a non-responsive and sympathetic position toward their aggravation experience. By developing care abilities, people can figure out how to notice torment sensations with more prominent composure, diminish profound reactivity and enduring, and work on their capacity to adapt to agony and uneasiness.

# End

All in all, integrative ways to deal with torment the board offer comprehensive techniques for tending to torment according to a complex point of view, enveloping the physical, profound, and mental parts of torment. By joining ordinary clinical therapies with correlative treatments, way of life mediations, and brain body rehearses, integrative agony the board approaches mean to advance recuperating, diminish torment, and work on generally speaking personal satisfaction for people with persistent agony conditions.

Integrative agony the board perceives torment as a complicated and multi-layered experience that requires an extensive and individualized way to deal with treatment. By tending to the basic reasons for torment, enabling patients to play a functioning job in their recuperating cycle, and cultivating joint effort among medical care suppliers from various disciplines, integrative methodologies can offer new roads for help with discomfort, mending, and prosperity.

As exploration keeps on developing, it is fundamental for keep investigating and refining integrative ways to deal with torment the board to upgrade results and improve the nature of care for people living with constant agony. By embracing an all-encompassing and patient-focused way to deal with torment the executives, we can all the more likely help people in their excursion toward recuperating, versatility, and reestablished prosperity.

# Chapter 14
# Case Studies and Success Stories

Contextual analyses and examples of overcoming adversity offer important bits of knowledge into the excursion of people who have defeated critical difficulties, accomplished their objectives, and changed their lives. From confronting ongoing ailments and handicaps to exploring individual battles and expert mishaps, these accounts feature the versatility, assurance, and tirelessness of people in conquering affliction and making progress. In this far reaching investigation, we dig into contextual analyses and examples of overcoming adversity from different areas, looking at the illustrations learned, procedures utilized, and key focus points for motivation and strengthening.

## *Understanding the Force of Contextual analyses and Examples of overcoming adversity*

Contextual investigations and examples of overcoming adversity give genuine instances of versatility, determination, and win over affliction. By sharing these accounts, people can track down motivation, trust, and inspiration to conquer their own difficulties and seek after their objectives with reestablished assurance and fortitude. Contextual analyses offer bits of knowledge into the techniques, outlook, and emotionally supportive networks that have added to progress, giving significant examples and direction to others confronting comparable battles.

# Contextual investigations from Various Spaces
# Wellbeing and Health:

## *Contextual investigation 1:*

## *Sarah's Excursion to Recuperation*

Sarah was determined to have a constant immune system condition that caused crippling aggravation, weakness, and versatility challenges. Regardless of the physical and profound cost of her sickness, not entirely set in stone to recover her wellbeing and prosperity. Through a blend of traditional clinical medicines, reciprocal treatments, and way of life changes, including dietary changes, stress the board strategies, and ordinary activity, Sarah bit by bit recaptured her solidarity, imperativeness, and feeling of direction. Today, Sarah is flourishing, dealing with her condition actually, and rousing others with her versatility and assurance to make every moment count.

## *Key Focus point:*

Sarah's process features the significance of tirelessness taking care of oneself, and an all-encompassing way to deal with wellbeing and health. By tending to the basic reasons for her disease and taking on an extensive treatment plan, Sarah had the option to conquer misfortune and accomplish ideal wellbeing and imperativeness.

# Self-improvement and Advancement:

## *Contextual analysis 2: John's Way to Individual Change*

John battled with low confidence, self-uncertainty, and apprehension about disappointment, which kept him away from seeking after his fantasies and objectives. Regardless of confronting various difficulties and snags en route, John stayed focused on his self-awareness and advancement venture. Through self-reflection, self-sympathy, and persistence, John slowly defeated his restricting convictions and got out of his usual range of familiarity to seek after his interests and yearnings. Today, John is flourishing in his profession, connections, and individual life, enabled by his freshly discovered certainty and flexibility.

## *Key Focal point:*

John's story outlines the groundbreaking force of mindfulness, self-acknowledgment, and tirelessness in conquering willful impediments and accomplishing self-improvement and satisfaction. By embracing change, facing challenges, and putting stock in himself, John had the option to rework his story and make a day to day existence lined up with his qualities and yearnings.

## Proficient Achievement:

## *Contextual investigation 3: Maria's Excursion to Innovative Achievement*

Maria confronted various difficulties and misfortunes on her pioneering venture, including monetary battles, market contest, and self-question. In spite of the snags, not set in stone to seek after her enthusiasm for social effect and development. Through versatility, creativity, and vital preparation, Maria explored the high points and low points of business, gaining from disappointments and misfortunes en route. Today, Maria's business is flourishing, having a beneficial outcome locally and then some, filled by her steady obligation to her vision and values.

## *Key Focal point:*

Maria's story epitomizes the significance of strength versatility, and constancy in making pioneering progress. By embracing difficulties as any open doors for development, learning, and advancement, Maria had the option to transform misfortunes into venturing stones toward her objectives and goals.

Examples of overcoming adversity from Assorted Foundations

# Defeating Incapacity:

## *Example of overcoming adversity 1: Alex's Excursion to Versatile Sports*

Alex was brought into the world with an innate incapacity that impacted his portability and actual capability. Regardless of the difficulties he confronted, Alex would not allow his inability to characterize him. Through versatile games, recovery treatments, and a steady local area, Alex found a freshly discovered feeling of strengthening, freedom, and reason. Today, Alex is a Paralympic competitor, moving others with his strength, assurance, and accomplishments on and off the field.

## *Key Focus point:*

Alex's example of overcoming adversity highlights the significance of strength, assurance, and flexibility in defeating handicap and accomplishing individual and athletic objectives. By embracing difficulties as any open doors for development and self-revelation, Alex changed affliction into win, demonstrating that the sky is the limit with diligence and assurance.

# Exploring Emotional well-being Difficulties:

## *Example of overcoming adversity 2: Emily's Excursion to Mental Wellbeing*

Emily battled with uneasiness, sadness, and low confidence, which influenced her own and proficient life. Regardless of the shame encompassing psychological sickness, Emily looked for help and backing from emotional wellness experts, peers, and friends and family. Through treatment, prescription, and taking care of oneself practices, Emily figured out how to deal with her side effects, develop self-empathy, and construct versatility despite affliction. Today, Emily is flourishing, upholding for psychological well-being mindfulness and supporting others on their excursion to health.

## *Key Action item:*

Emily's example of overcoming adversity features the significance of looking for help, ending the quiet encompassing psychological sickness, and rehearsing taking care of oneself and self-empathy. By focusing on emotional well-being and looking for help when required, Emily had the option to defeat difficulties and recover her prosperity and feeling of direction.

# End

Taking everything into account, contextual investigations and examples of overcoming adversity offer strong stories of strength, assurance, and win over difficulty. Whether beating wellbeing challenges, seeking after self-awareness and advancement, making proficient progress, or exploring handicap and emotional well-being battles, these accounts rouse trust,  inspiration, and strengthening in others confronting comparative difficulties.

By sharing our accounts of flexibility and change, we make a far reaching influence of motivation and strengthening, reminding others that they are in good company in their battles and that recuperating and development are conceivable, even notwithstanding difficulty. Through tirelessness, boldness, and backing, people can revamp their accounts, conquer hindrances, and make lives loaded up with reason, enthusiasm, and satisfaction.

# Chapter 15
# The Future of Flexibility and Pain Reduction

As we look forward to the fate of adaptability and torment decrease, we imagine a scene described by continuous progressions, developments, and arising patterns that hold the commitment of changing how we get it, approach, and oversee outer muscle wellbeing and torment. From state of the art advances and logical disclosures to developing treatment modalities and all-encompassing methodologies, the eventual fate of adaptability and agony decrease is ready to reform medical care, upgrade patient results, and work on personal satisfaction for millions around the world. In this far reaching investigation, we dig into the key patterns, improvements, and potential outcomes molding the fate of adaptability and torment decrease.

## Bridling Innovation for Customized Care

The joining of innovation into medical care holds gigantic potential for upsetting the manner in which we approach adaptability and agony decrease. Progressions in wearable gadgets, advanced wellbeing stages, and telemedicine are empowering customized, remote, and constant observing of outer muscle wellbeing, considering early identification of issues and proactive mediations. Wearable sensors and savvy articles of clothing outfitted with movement following capacities can give significant experiences into development examples, act, and biomechanics, enabling people to upgrade their adaptability and forestall injury.

Besides, tile-restoration and virtual exercise based recuperation stages are making outer muscle care more available and advantageous, permitting patients to get customized treatment and direction from the solace of their homes. These advances work with remote observing, virtual counsels, and intuitive activity programs custom fitted to individual necessities, upgrading consistence, commitment, and results for patients recuperating from wounds or overseeing persistent agony conditions.

# Accuracy Medication and Biomarkers

The development of accuracy medication and
Biomarker-based approaches holds guarantee for altering the analysis, treatment, and the executives of outer muscle conditions and torment. Accuracy medication means to fit treatment systems to the singular qualities, hereditary qualities, and inclinations of every patient, upgrading restorative results and limiting secondary effects. By utilizing progressed imaging methods, hereditary profiling, and biomarker investigation, clinicians can distinguish customized risk factors, anticipate treatment reactions, and foster designated intercessions for outer muscle problems.

Biomarkers, like fiery markers, hereditary variations, and atomic marks, offer significant experiences into the basic components of torment and irritation, directing the advancement of novel therapeutics and mediations. By distinguishing explicit biomarkers related with torment awareness, tissue harm, or aggravation, specialists can foster more exact analytic apparatuses, prognostic pointers, and designated treatments for outer muscle conditions, prompting more compelling agony the board procedures and worked on understanding results.

# Regenerative Medication and Tissue Designing

The field of regenerative medication and tissue designing holds guarantee for changing the treatment of outer muscle wounds and degenerative circumstances by tackling the body's normal mending instruments to fix and recover harmed tissues. Progresses in undeveloped cell treatment, platelet-rich plasma (PRP) treatment, and tissue designing procedures are empowering the improvement of creative methodologies for upgrading tissue fix, decreasing irritation, and advancing recovery in harmed or unhealthy tissues.

Immature microorganism treatments, got from different sources like bone marrow, fat tissue, or umbilical rope blood, have shown guarantee in advancing tissue recovery and lessening torment in conditions like osteoarthritis, ligament wounds, and spinal string wounds. Essentially, PRP treatment, which includes infusing concentrated platelets and development factors into harmed tissues, has shown viability in diminishing torment, further developing capability, and advancing tissue recuperating in outer muscle problems.

Tissue designing methodologies, for example, 3D bio printing and platform based treatments, empower the manufacture of redone tissue develops that copy the construction and capability of local tissues. These designed tissues can be utilized for fixing harmed ligament, tendons, or ligaments, giving a regenerative answer for outer muscle wounds and degenerative circumstances. By tackling the regenerative capability of immature microorganisms, development factors, and biomaterials, regenerative medication offers new roads for tending to the hidden reasons for agony and brokenness, preparing for additional powerful and strong medicines.

# Integrative and All-encompassing Methodologies

Notwithstanding mechanical and biomedical headways, the fate of adaptability and torment decrease is described by a developing acknowledgment of the significance of integrative and comprehensive methodologies that address the interconnectedness of the psyche, body, and soul. Integrative modalities like yoga, needle therapy, knead treatment, and care based rehearses are earning respect as successful adjunctive treatments for overseeing torment, diminishing pressure, and advancing generally speaking prosperity.

These methodologies stress the significance of tending to the basic mental, profound, and way of life factors that add to agony and brokenness, considering the singular's one of a kind bio-psychosocial setting. By consolidating mind-body methods, stress the board techniques, and way of life changes into treatment plans, clinicians can engage patients to play a functioning job in their mending cycle and develop versatility, mindfulness, and taking care of oneself practices that help long haul torment the executives and health.

## Patient-Focused Care and Shared Direction

The fate of adaptability and torment decrease is portrayed by a shift toward patient-focused care models that focus on joint effort, correspondence, and shared decision production among patients and medical services suppliers. Perceiving that every patient is novel and may have various objectives, values, and inclinations
 Patient-focused care accentuates dynamic commitment, sympathy, and association in the restorative relationship.

Shared direction includes a cooperative cycle where patients and suppliers cooperate to settle on informed conclusions about treatment choices, considering the patient's inclinations, values, and objectives, as well as the most ideal that anyone could hope to find proof and clinical mastery. By including patients in direction and co-planning treatment designs that line up with their singular necessities and needs, clinicians can improve patient fulfillment, adherence, and results, encouraging a feeling of strengthening, independence, and confidence in the remedial relationship.

# End

All in all, the eventual fate of adaptability and torment decrease is portrayed by a combination of mechanical, biomedical, and all-encompassing methodologies that hold guarantee for changing outer muscle care and working on tolerant results. From bridling the force of innovation for customized checking and remote consideration to utilizing accuracy medication and regenerative treatments for designated mediations, the fate of agony the executives is set apart by development, joint effort, and patient-focused care.

By embracing progressions in innovation, biomedical exploration, and integrative modalities, medical care suppliers can upgrade adaptability and agony decrease systems, tailor therapy ways to deal with individual necessities, and enable patients to play a functioning job in their recuperating venture. As we keep on propelling comprehension we might interpret outer muscle wellbeing and agony, we are ready to open additional opportunities for upgrading personal satisfaction, advancing health, and further developing results for people living with torment.

9 798324 881511